RAFT

Anne Gill helped found the Second City Poets, a Birmingham based collective whose show, *Playground*, was commissioned for the Verve Poetry Festival. She has performed at events in the UK and abroad, and was a part of the University of Birmingham's winning UniSlam team in 2018. Her work has appeared in print in various places including *Strix*, *Ink Sweat and Tears*, and anthology, *The Dizziness of Freedom*. She is a submissions reader for Bare Fiction, and was shortlisted for the 2018 Outspoken Prize for Poetry. She is currently in Newcastle where she is studying her Masters and becoming friends with various cats on the way to work.

Raft

Published by Bad Betty Press in 2019
www.badbettypress.com

Cover design by Amy Acre

Printed and bound in the United Kingdom

A CIP record of this book is available from the British Library.

ISBN: 978-1-9997147-7-2

raft

ANNE GILL

BAD BETTY
PRESS

It is not only the moment of the event, but of the passing out of it that is traumatic; that survival itself, in other words, can be a crisis.

– Cathy Caruth

Contents

When the man came
into me the birds sang in the trees
and, in the park, children screamed.

Across the ocean my mother told my father
that she loved him, and my father's tongue twisted
into chaffinches when he said it back.

When the man came, a dog caught a ball
and refused to give it back
and ice creaked under the weight.

Cars rushed by and toppled
into each other and a woman, waiting by the lights,
listened to a podcast on neurotransmitters.

A ship crossed the ocean
with dried goods and flood defences were
rooted into place as the man came into me.

When the man came,
his hands were soft and sharp
and his eyes were there.

When the man came,
my body, holding an ocean inside of it,
craved drowning, or camouflage,
or algae.

Raft

Clouds: A Scientific Study

Convection is vital in the production of cumulonimbus clouds. Warm air and cold air move about, taking turns in different positions. It is rather like a penguin huddle where penguins take turns in the middle and when they are warm are moved to the edge. The huddle takes a lot of energy and so does a cumulonimbus cloud. Cumulonimbus clouds are the energy equivalent of 100,000 penguins.

> Two penguins sit opposite each other playing chess.
>
> 'Your turn,' says Penguin 1.

The air in a cumulonimbus cloud is unstable and turbulent. No matter how much the air mixes it does not homogenise. Penguin 2 is going to lose at chess.

> 'I said your turn.
>
> Hurry up, I'm getting bored.'

The cumulonimbus cloud has grown so tall it has hit the top of the troposphere and started growing outwards. Penguin 2 is stuck against the ceiling of the troposphere.

> 'Move something.'
>
> 'I can't.'
>
> 'You have to.'

Ivy

The seal twists about
inside of us like a creeper.
Rushes into arms and head,
tells us we can never
escape, that it will be like this
forever. The seal licks his lips,
slaps his arse and threatens death.

Later, Penguin 2 gardens, rips
down ivy from the side of the house
and the green sap runs like blood
and sticks in his feathers
with the sound of the seal's voice:
I love you, you want this, you need this.

When the ivy is stuffed
into gardening bins and spills
onto the pavement
scars remain on the house.
We cannot get rid of them.

Playground Games

At school Penguin 2's son falls
in the playground and has to have
his wing clicked back into place
and put in a sling.

On the way back from the hospital
Penguin 2 drives over a pothole
and his son cries. Penguin 2 is
exhausted.

It is Penguin 2's fault for driving
over the pothole and hurting his son
~~his son would be better~~
~~off without him~~

he won't stop crying.

TV Dinner

They sit
not touching
in front of Happy Feet
and ice cream.

Swaddled in painkillers
Penguin 2's son watches
a pothole through the window.

Pandora

In the middle of a panic attack
Penguin 2 vomits

up four kinds of fish
seaweed
three perfectly spherical ice cubes
a toenail
five rolls of cling film wrapped
around lungs.

All he is left with is a toy truck
with a chip to the rear.

Unravel

We keep seeing their faces at night:
mind plays then runs in technicolour.
I remember there was a lamp, blue, on my right.

We keep seeing his face at night
in high definition. Tape catches, unravels –
he's like a VHS tape, jammed in, not right.

You remember there was a lamp, blue, on your right.
remember the [↺] you remember the –
the shadows are him in our rooms at night.

We keep seeing their faces at night
we keep seeing [‖]
they hold our minds in theirs hands; squeeze too tight.

I remember there was a lamp, blue, on my right.
I remember [◄◄] you remember [◄◄] –
I remember headlights.

I keep seeing his – keep
feeling his [↺] we can't stop can't stop
seeing their faces at night.
I remember there was a lamp, blue, on my right.

Solid Ground

Here is a sachet of sugar, a wooden spoon,
it is recyclable.

Here is a bin, a paper cup
bent in two.

Here is a keypad, a door,
here is solid ground.

Here is a plastic chair and a jacket
thin as lined paper.

Here is a bin bag.
Here there are voices.

Here there are always voices,
the words are recycled.

Here is a body.
It is reduced.

Cannon Hill Park

Trees curve in
to hold you;

blue branches
scratch at cheeks

and the leaves
are yellow in your hair.

Grass moves
as the sea

sways then
swallows you

'til you inhale
pink blades.

The trees breathe loudly.
You taste iron.

You Have to Cancel

the cat is planning a coup a tarantula broke in and is holding you
hostage you spilt baked beans over everything you own you should
probably clean it up you have to cancel your soft toy woke up you're
hosting a funeral your pot plant died you can't leave the house in
case a wasp flies in and no one's around to let it out

Green Trauma Bear

At the clinic they give out green trauma bears. *This will make you feel safe.* The green trauma bears are silent and green and have sharp claws encased in bubble wrap to stop accidents. The green trauma bears are gentle and dusty. They are about half the size of a lamp post. It is understood that they will help. It is understood that *this will make you feel safe.*

Subject 1 exhibits symptoms of anxiety when walking down the road at night even though a green trauma bear follows, plodding methodically at a safe distance. Subject 2 does not seem to notice its green trauma bear and Subject 3 pops all the bubbles on the bubble wrap, holds the green trauma bear's paw in place and scores their arm along the claws. The green trauma bear sighs and does not react. The green trauma bear is just doing its job which, quite frankly, it is not prepared for.

The green trauma bear must follow the Subject wherever it goes like a shadow. The Subject does not feel safe. The Subject does not feel safe. Subject 12 uses a green trauma bear as a ladder to scale the fence by the railway line before implanting itself on the track. A green trauma bear follows like a concerned parent. A green trauma bear follows like a shadow. A green trauma bear follows even though it would probably rather be playing pool right now. A green trauma bear follows.

Penguin 2 Is Told to Write a Gratitude Journal

I saw a cow
out of everyone else the cow chose to chase me out of everyone else
the cow chased me and gave me free cardio
out of everyone else the cow chased me and I fell in cow shit and a
bird shat on my head and
that's good luck out of everyone else I got good luck
I bought a sandwich with my good luck
I bought a cheese sandwich with my good luck and it didn't have
much cheese in it which is good
because some people are lactose intolerant I got a very plain very dry
sandwich with my good luck
and it meant I drank water and I should drink more water I am
grateful for water
I got sandwich crumbs everywhere and I am grateful for the mice
I always wanted a pet and one day they just showed up I can't leave
the house without panicking which is good
because now I can start a diet and I can't do anything
without having a panic attack and I am grateful because it engages
my core
I am grateful that I can't stop remembering the rape at the time
of the rape I was wearing old clothes I am grateful I was probably
going to throw them out anyway I am grateful that I shower more

and I am grateful for cleanliness and I am grateful that he didn't
kill me and I am grateful that it only happened once and and I am
grateful that it didn't happen to my son I am grateful that it didn't
happen to my son I am so grateful that it didn't happen to my son

Saturday

Penguin 2 visits the city farm where pigs are fed bananas dripping in chocolate and a cow cries because it has no water and Penguin 2 doesn't help it. They stare at each other until Penguin 2 says *I want to die* and the cow cries for water and Penguin 2 says *I mean it* and the cow drools on Penguin 2's feet until he leaves.

Pembrokeshire

When Penguin 2 dives
headfirst off the cliff's edge
and into the puddle of rocks below
his son is building houses out of Lego.

Only, when Penguin 2 dives
headfirst off the cliff's edge
towards the full stop below,
he doesn't actually dive.

Instead, he stands, feet curved
and loving over the cliff's edge
and thinks about sentence ends;
methane ballooning out

of permafrost, and his son, who rocks
on plastic chairs and is rubbing out
the right answers. And time has the
decency to retreat on its lunch break

as Penguin 2 cradles
the sandstone with his feet
until his son takes root on a bench
and the school calls asking where he is.

Penguin 2 apologises, steps back,
and returns to the car.

Dandelion

Before we tried to kill ourselves we tap-danced
to the rhythm of the extractor fan and the out
breaths of dandelions. We made tea
from their roots and neglected to wash off the dirt.

We ate all our favourite foods; mash
with smiley-faced potatoes and Penguin bars
on the side, but this still didn't cheer us up.
We cried by the window for dramatic effect.

We left the front door unlocked, gave the cat
plenty of food so it wouldn't have to stuff
itself full of us. We did a test run with Aldi
razors to see what it was like and part of us wanted to

chicken out. Before we tried to kill ourselves
we told the lady at the doctor's office
who didn't believe we really meant it, and told us
to practice breathing when we got home.

We made a pros and cons list and the only things
on the cons list were that we were scared and
our mothers would yell at us if we failed.
We decided to do it on Monday.

And while the pills danced in our stomachs
our mothers visited and made us talk to our grandparents
about slippers and the pills were putting pinpricks in our faces
and we were so excited that our hearts were beating

out rhythms of the screaming dandelions we boiled
and drank and didn't even have the decency to wash.
And we went to sleep in our rooms, hearts screeching
and didn't think about how much we hated ourselves.

Bluebell

You can only smell the grass when you take out your gum and press
it into an old tissue. There's a motorway underlaid
with the sound of a bird and from where you're sitting
you can see the tower blocks of the north. Someone rides an electric
bike through the field and you wonder if, far off, someone is mowing
their lawn, hunched over and nodding to themselves.

It's warmer outside than in your flat and here the dogs talk to you.
They tell you how water bottles bounce better than sticks,
and about the hundreds of smells contained in a single patch
of grass; and you tell them that you can't see shapes
in the clouds anymore, and that sometimes you're scared
there's a person in your shadow you can't quite touch.

And a dog holds its wet nose to your wrist and is silent
and you tell it that sometimes it feels like you've been left
in the supermarket and everyone's at home enjoying hot tea
and freshly made cake (probably rainbow or red velvet
because those are your favourites) and no one has noticed
that they left you, or where they left you, and the bread
in the bread aisle is stale and hard when you touch it.

The dogs just sit there as you try not to think about the cows
grazing nearby. You remember one of the cows grooming the other
and the length of its tongue as it ran its sandpaper through the fur of
its companion, and the delicacy of it and you want
your mother to stop forcing you to hug her and you want
to sit in a corner where you can see everything.

And the dogs are breathing regularly. You just want them,
and the cows in their strength to stand around you, the cows
breathing their grassy breaths on you. And you don't want anyone
to touch you. You want the doctors to believe you
when you say you're unwell; you're so terrified of the scales
in your house and the pills you're studiously not counting
and you just want the cows to chew. To allow you to nestle into them
for a moment. To tell you that you're here.

Fairground

His son holds his arms in the air
sling empty on his chest,
head tilted to the sky.

When the ride stops
Penguin 2 ruffles the feathers
on his son's head.

And the seal still itches
his brain into an ache
that leans over bridges

and into medicine cabinets
but it is less often now.
Some days, he imagines

music swelling to his step.
David Attenborough's voice
swimming over it.

They leave with ice lollies
dripping around them, arguing
over who was better at bumper cars.

Acknowledgements

Thank you to everyone who has ever let me overshare. Who has walked me, or has walked their friends, home. Who sends *did you get home safe?* texts.

To the Birmingham poetry community, the UniSlam community, the Second City Poets.

To the editors of *Closed Gates or Open Arms?* and *The Dizziness of Freedom* for publishing 'Dandelion' and 'Green Trauma Bear' in their original forms.

My teachers, particularly Mr Hancock and Luke Kennard.

To those who have been supportive of my work: especially Leon Priestnall and Stuart Bartholomew.

Those who inspire me to write better, and who have taught me the value of openness. Toby Campion, Sean Colletti, Jess Davies, Jasmine Gardosi, Nafeesa Hamid, Emily Harrison, Kieran Hayes, Shaun Hill, Hannah Ledlie, Kadie Newman, Hannah Swingler.

Nafeesa Hamid and Antosh Wojcik: thank you for your kind words.

My friends and family. My mum, Benjamin and Jane. To Tom and Abby who, without fail, get me out of bed in the morning. And to my number one drinking partners, Alex Hamzij and Emma Thompson.

The NHS, Maria, and RSVP Birmingham.

The boys who let me share their taxi. The man at Kings Cross who gave me water in the middle of a panic attack. The lady at the corner shop who gave me a drink when I didn't have the money.

Jake Wild Hall and Amy Acre. Amy, thanks for asking the right questions of my writing, and for listening. I am indebted to you and your work.

Sean Colletti, for dancing with me and putting up with mosquitoes, for listening and calling the doctors when I couldn't, and for cooking maybe the best breakfasts out there.

Other titles by Bad Betty Press

Solomon's World
Jake Wild Hall

TIGER
Rebecca Tamás

Unremember
Joel Auterson

The Death of a Clown
Tom Bland

In My Arms
Setareh Ebrahimi

While I Yet Live
Gboyega Odubanjo

The Story Is
Kate B Hall

The Dizziness Of Freedom
Edited by Amy Acre
and Jake Wild Hall

I'm Shocked
Iris Colomb

Ode to Laura Smith
Aischa Daughtery

The Pale Fox
Katie Metcalfe

Lightning Source UK Ltd.
Milton Keynes UK
UKHW041527250420
362197UK00002B/246

9 781999 714772